THE ART OF YOGA

In a nutshell, yoga is a powerful art form.

It's basically a form of meditation, used to explore the inner self and to connect to your higher self. It's very often used to help you connect with your spirit, connect with your other true self or soul.

In yoga, you are given a list of affirmations, when used properly, they encourage your mind to become more awake, and to be more aware of everything that is going on, in your body, mind, and your environment. It's like a self-coaching session, where you take full, positive conscious responsibility for your own future and develop and increase the power to act in accordance with your own true self.

Regular practice of this type of art has been shown to have a very strong and positive effect on the body and the mind. It's also been shown to improve your reaction time, your physical strength, your energy, your balance, your breathing, and your ability to focus. The power of Yoga can be applied to a number of things like weight loss, muscle strengthening, joint rehabilitation, detoxification, and many other positive life-affirming changes. Yoga is very simple to build upon and provides great life-changing rewards in return.

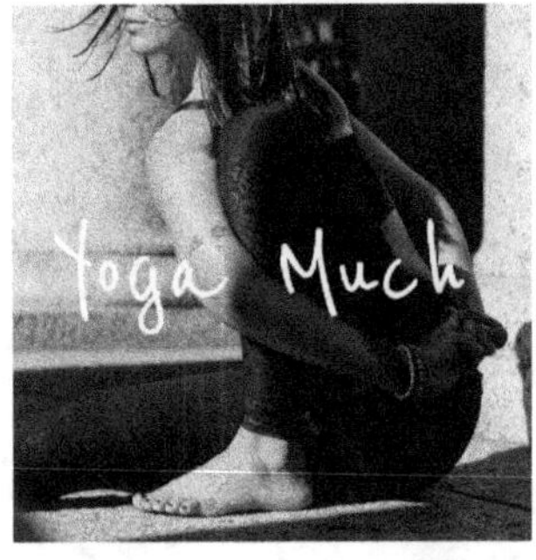

When you first begin, we encourage you to spend 5 minutes working on the poses of your choice, it's then good practice to spend 10 minutes lying down, and then you spend 15 minutes going into the "manas" or void and "being in the moment".

During these sessions, you have the opportunity to connect emotionally and physically to your higher self. Yoga when done properly produce very strong self-connected experiences. It can create a very strong sense of empowerment as you work to bring your body and mind into alignment, through the use of specific poses and exercises. The benefits of yoga are obvious: Over time you will gain improved posture, greater overall health, increased flexibility, better immunity, and strength, decreased stress, increased creativity, enhanced willpower, and confidence, which are positive benefits that we can all use on a daily basis.

The key to maintaining and building upon the benefits providing in yoga is a regular practice. For instance, doing 5 minutes of Vinyasa (the process of stringing postures together), every day for about 5 days in a row will create a number of health benefits, such as improved attitude, positive spirit and mood increase, better concentration, and your focus improvement. Other benefits include decreasing your blood pressure, anxiety, tension, and your heart rate while increasing your body temperature, oxygen intake, metabolic heart rate, production of endorphins, and levels of GABA. All of which when combined and repeated daily, contribute to the better quality of life and health we all seek.

One of the things I find fascinating about yoga is that people can do this every day with great compounding benefits. The poses that are offered with yoga practice offer a pretty wide range of choices. You can choose to either practice with these standard yoga poses or you can do your own poses. Overall, If you want to get into yoga or purify your body in any way, whether it's for a short time or for a long time, it's really hard to find a system or exercise to do, which offers better benefits to your long term mental, emotional or physical health than this. This book will focus and concentrate on several ways to practice yoga and demonstrate poses through verse and images.

We will touch on Vinyasa, Hatha, Kundalini, Ashtanga, Bikram, Yin, Restorative, and Anusara yoga practices and poses. Then visit several other popular yoga practices as well. Welcome to yoga as an art form.

UNDERSTANDING YOGA

Before we dive into learning some of the great yoga poses, exercises, and practices, it's very important for you to understand, what yoga is, some of its most common practices, and why it's so wildly popular around the world as a form of stress relief, mood booster, pain management, exercise and more.

In order to gain a better understanding of the different yoga types such as Vinyasa, Hatha, Kundalini, Ashtanga, Bikram, Yin, Restorative, and Anusara we must first define them, and then provide a brief explanation through a series of questions and answers listing the benefits of each yoga type on the human body both mentally, physically and spiritually.

Let's talk **VINYASA.**

Question: What is Vinyasa?

Answer: A vinyasa is a smooth transition between asanas in

styles of modern yoga.

Vinya is the first of the four foundations of yoga: it is the science of the senses and of thought. It aims at developing the mind, as well as the body and soul. For this reason, it is sometimes called the foundation of yoga, and the science of self-inquiry, as it aims directly at the development of intelligence.

Vinyasa delves directly into the sense media of sight, sound, and smell. These are studied, developed, and refined to the point where they become the vehicle for the soul. The senses are developed until they are no longer he determinant factor in thought, but rather they are the vehicle for the soul to receive information.

Next, **HATHA.**

Question: What is Hatha?

Answer: Is a branch of yoga that means (force) and a system of physical techniques.

In the process of this practice, the practitioner uses the special leg posture called the Baddha Konasana. In addition to being one of the poses that are commonly found in the Hatha series.

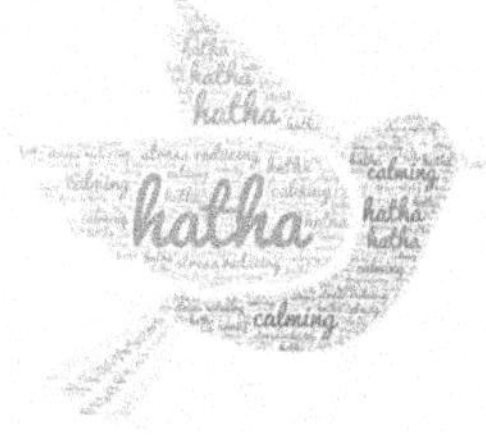

HATHA

the Baddha Konasana is another pose that is very useful in calming the mind and reducing stress. Because of this fact, this posture is commonly incorporated into the lessons of this form of yoga.

And now, **KUNDALINI**.

Question: What is Kundalini?

Answer: Is the release of energy through specific meditation and yoga practice.

It is believed that Kundalini uses energy which is derived from the direct line of energy from the tops of our heads and straight down through the bottom of our spine.

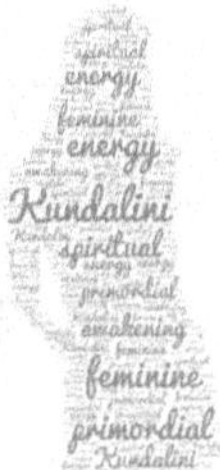

KUNDALINI

When this energy is engaged, it is said that we humans are able to create an energy flow upward through our bodies from the base of our spines towards our heads, which in turn creates a spiritual balance of energy throughout our bodies.

Kundalini is directly associated with a divine awakened feminine primordial energy within the yoga community.

On to, **ASHTANGA**.

Question: What is Ashtanga?

Answer: An energetic style of synchronized breathing with movements in yoga practice.

Ashtanga directly translated means the eight-limbed practice one would use on the path to achieving the state of yoga which is also known by the name of Samadhi.

ASHTANGA

Ashtanga yoga may be perfect for the beginner since most sequences are short and allow the beginner to really move at their own pace.

The pace of changing poses and breathing techniques can also be slowed so that the beginner can learn each pose precisely at their own pace.

The very popular, **BIKRAM**.

Question: What is Bikram?

Answer: A hot yoga of 26 specific postures practiced in a room heated to 105 degrees.

Bikram is an exercise system of hot yoga, which consists of 26 sequenced postures, practiced in a room heated to 105 °F. Bikram yoga is very demanding with each program lasting 90-minutes and is not for the faint of heart and is not recommended for the beginner.

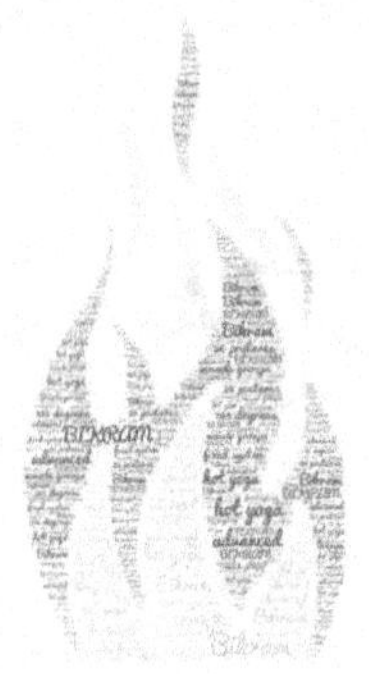

Bikram yoga involves different stretching and standing poses that encourage concentrated, forceful contractions of your body's major muscle groups. Again this prolonged yoga activity is very demanding and is designed to raise your heart rate and thoroughly exercise your major muscle groups to exhaustion.

The very popular and oft-discussed Yin, Restorative, and Anusara yoga styles will be further explained and detailed later in the book through visual images and discussions.

WHY CHOOSE YOGA

The main reason for choosing yoga is simply for the tremendous mental, physical, and spiritual health benefits yoga when used as a daily practice provides.

Yoga when practiced regularly keeps your body and mind healthy not only physically, but mentally as well. Yoga helps us create positive breathing habits, and by developing good breathing habits you can strengthen your back and neck muscles, which promotes good posture, while controlled inhaling and exhaling is the heartbeat of your body. Proper breathing maintains your health and helps your mind to remain calm. A good mind keeps you healthy.

A bad mind can lead you to unhealthy situations and can even cause you harm. The good thing about yoga and its breathing exercises is that there is no need for pills or medicines and is 100% healthy for you with no side effects.

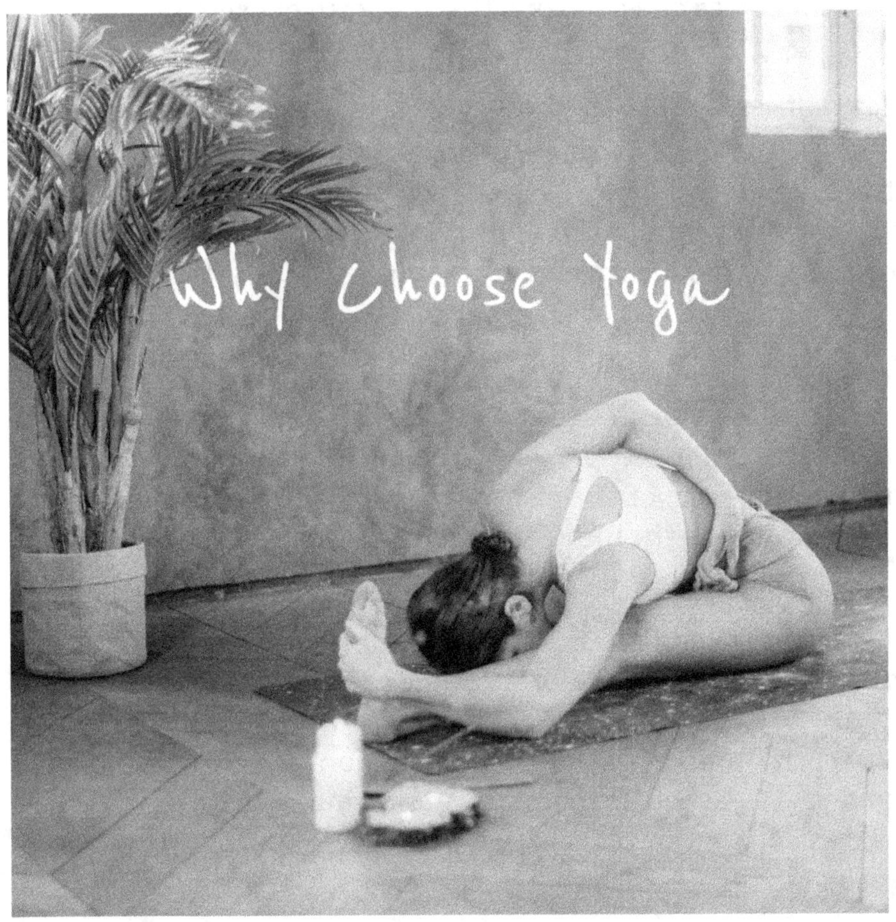

image edits RyPul Media

Yoga will give you clarity of thought. Yoga, in general, is about controlling your breathing, with clearness of mind is being the desired result of this form of exercise.

The best thing about it is that this is a lifelong endeavor that you can enjoy and practice whenever you desire. You will notice over time that you will be able to think clearly right after completing a yoga regime. Many people experience significant and important positive life-changing mental and physical advantages when they commit to yoga as a daily practice and form of exercise.

Yoga will give you a sense of balance and strength. Although beautiful in form, yoga is a physical workout, which greatly strengthens the body, soul, and mind. One thing that is not mentioned in much information is that it is also about maintaining balance in everything you do.

Yoga helps to build endurance and the ability to maintain your perfect balance in all aspects of your life. And for those people who have been inactive for a period of time in their lives, yoga is an excellent form of exercise to help you get moving again while helping you take the mind off things for a little bit.

Yoga will give you an overall feeling of peace. Remember peace or the sense of peace, is not the same as happiness. Peace is about staying in a position without injuring yourself. It is about staying in a position and maintaining a position. It can also be about looking at a particular spot without moving. When you are able to create a position and stay in that position, the chances are you will feel better.

Yoga will help you heal.

As millions of people around the world will attest to, yogasana, or downward-facing dog, will help your health to heal. It is about keeping your spine straight and your back straight. These are movements that will help you to keep your spine, and your back, straight. There will be a little bit of twisting and curving.

Many people will try to do this as a gymnastic exercise and find this to be quite challenging, but if you take the time to do it at least once a week, you will notice a lot of improvement. For many people, twisting and curving will help their back pain.

So, there are many ways to take the mind off the pain. You can take the mind off pain with regular hard work, with stretching your spine, with yoga, with a few minutes of gentle stretching, or with meditation. Each of these takes the mind off the pain and can help you heal.

Remember the number one priority, and that will take the mind off pain is having overall good health. With yoga, you can enjoy the process of getting your body and your spirit back to normal.

THE HOW OF YOGA

The purpose of yoga is to calm the mind and to help the practitioner focus on the internal energy that is within them. To be more specific, the purpose of yoga postures and poses is to take your mind to the inner self through intelligent guidance.

The term "intelligently" seems to be lost in translation among people who may not know much about yoga. While the term "inner self" refers to the energy that is contained within our bodies and the term "intelligently" refers to our level of understanding within the practice of yoga. It is said within yoga circles that once you understand the intelligence contained within you, you then understand the intelligence of your body and the capacity it has to transform you mentally, physically, and spiritually with yoga.

When you practice yoga, it is important to be at ease with your breathing. The purpose of mastering breath control is to be able to get you in touch with the energy that is within you and to be able to utilize it in order to achieve a higher level of consciousness. There is a tendency to push the limits of your body and to push yourself physically and emotionally, and it is important that you be careful not to push yourself too far, too fast.

It is suggested that you practice the yoga poses for a maximum of 10 minutes, but no more than 20 minutes. If you practice the posture for 20 minutes or more, it is highly recommended that you include one or two rounds of ab work for proper energy balance.

Yoga will help give your body structure and balance that is both powerful and refined, and when you begin to practice yoga regularly, you will also learn that it is much you can learn about your own physical and emotional needs.

You may be able to refine your ability to focus and focus your mind on one thing for a longer period of time. You may also be able to develop a greater capacity to concentrate when you are frustrated or angry, or you may be able to become more adept at remaining calm and composed in the face of frustration and anger. You may also be able to learn how to get more organized and to have a greater ability to stay organized.

Remember a very important part of yoga is meditation. It includes focusing on a specific area of the body in order to improve the health of that area. The breathing pattern while meditating is also an important aspect of doing it correctly.

Also, proper breathing while doing a yoga posture is an important aspect of gaining the maximum benefit of the yoga exercise you have engaged in. With any luck, the practice of yoga will help you develop your capacity to remain focused in the face of stress and to help you get more organized and to feel less stressed when you placed in difficult situations.

BEST 10 YOGA POSES

Now that we have explained yoga as an art form, provided some great background on yoga and its history, defined why you should make yoga a daily part of your routine life, and told you "how to yoga", its now time to give you the top 10 power poses and postures to help transform your life starting today.

I have selected poses that will be great for the mind, body, and spirit, and, these poses are great for beginners and advanced students as well. I encourage you to take a few minutes each day to practice my "best 10" yoga poses, which are certain to improve your mind, body, and spirit.

These power poses are certain to get your day started by providing a positive boost of adrenaline, good spiritual energy, and long-lasting energetic mental balance.

Number One

THE DOWNWARD FACING DOG (AKA) Adho Mukha Svanasana

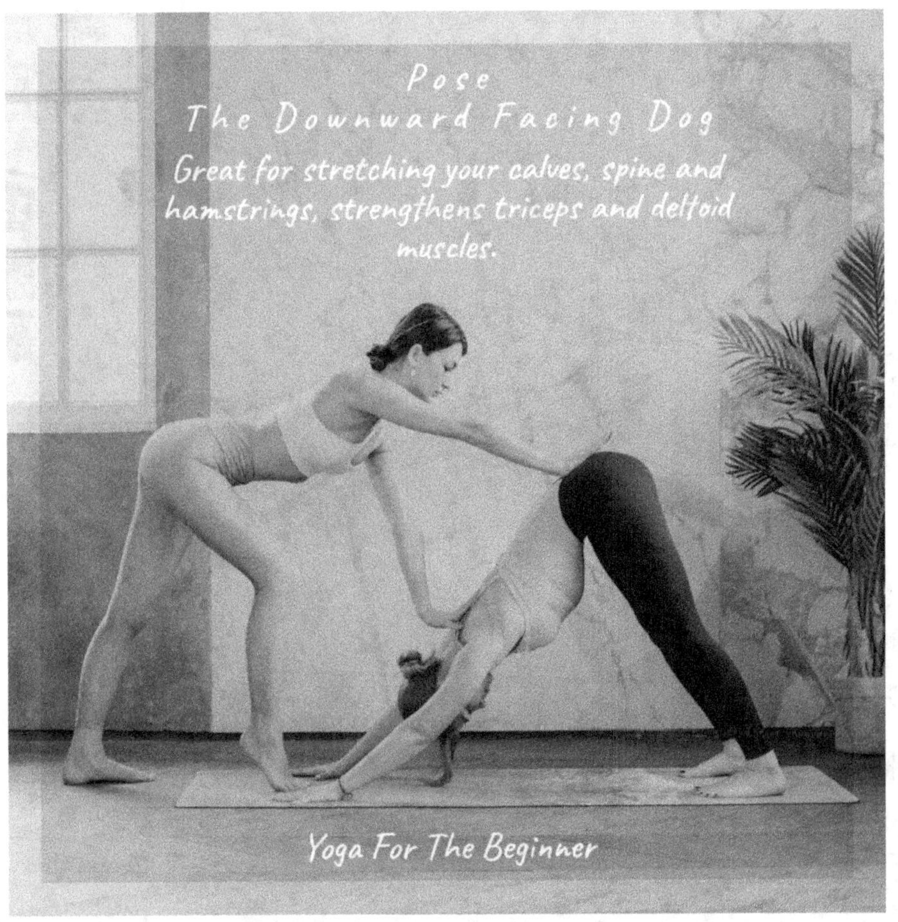

THE DOWNWARD FACING DOG - (AKA) Adho Mukha Svanasana

Number Two

THE CAMEL POSE - (AKA) Ustrasana

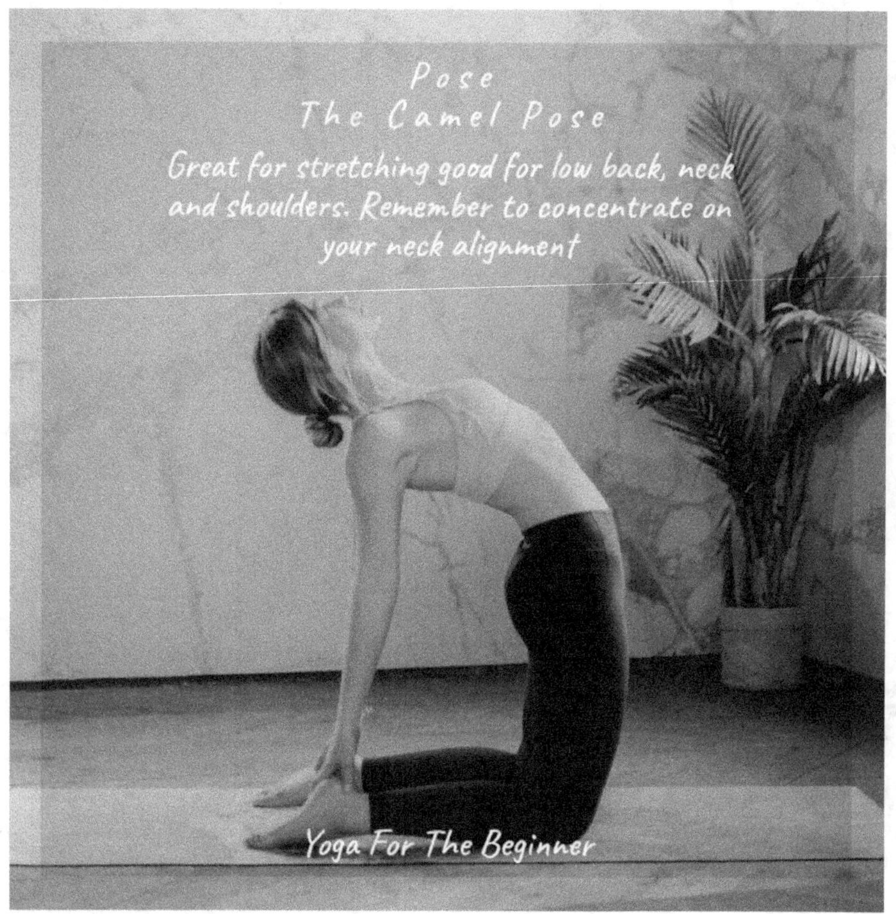

THE CAMEL POSE - (AKA) Ustrasana

Number Three

THE COW FACE POSE - (AKA) Gomukhasana

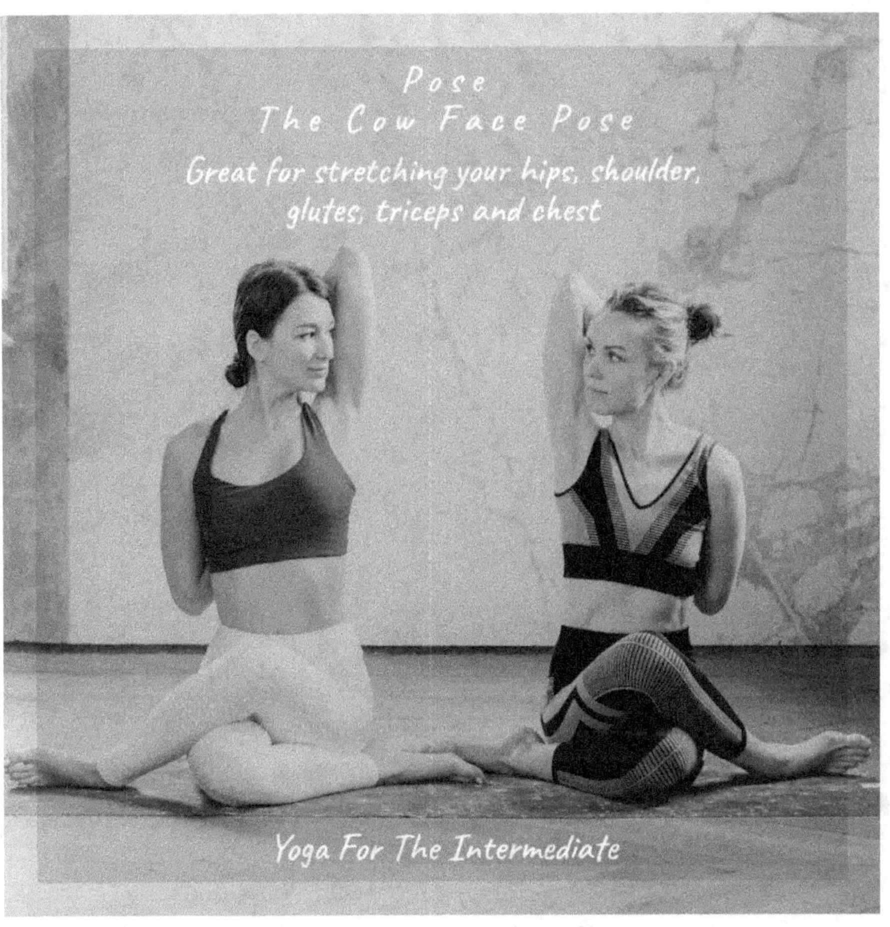

THE COW FACE POSE - (AKA) Gomukhasana

Number Four

THE CORPSE POSE - (AKA) Savasana

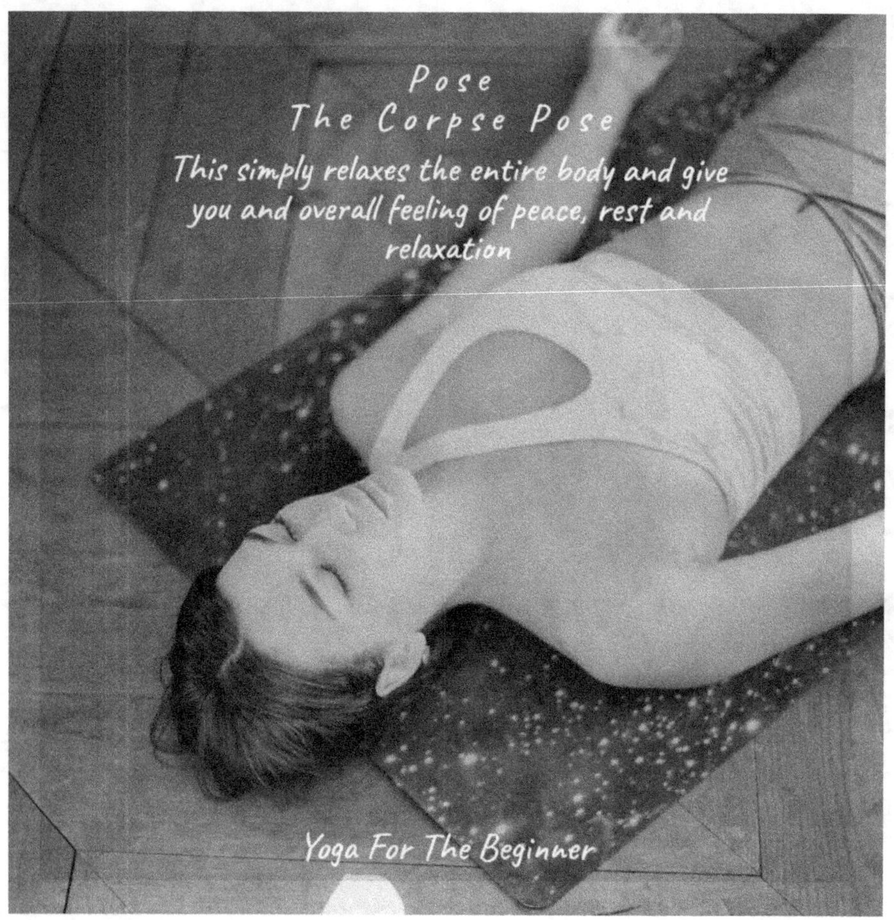

THE CORPSE POSE - (AKA) Savasana

Number Five

THE FOUR LIMBED STAFF POSE - (AKA) Chaturanga Dandasana

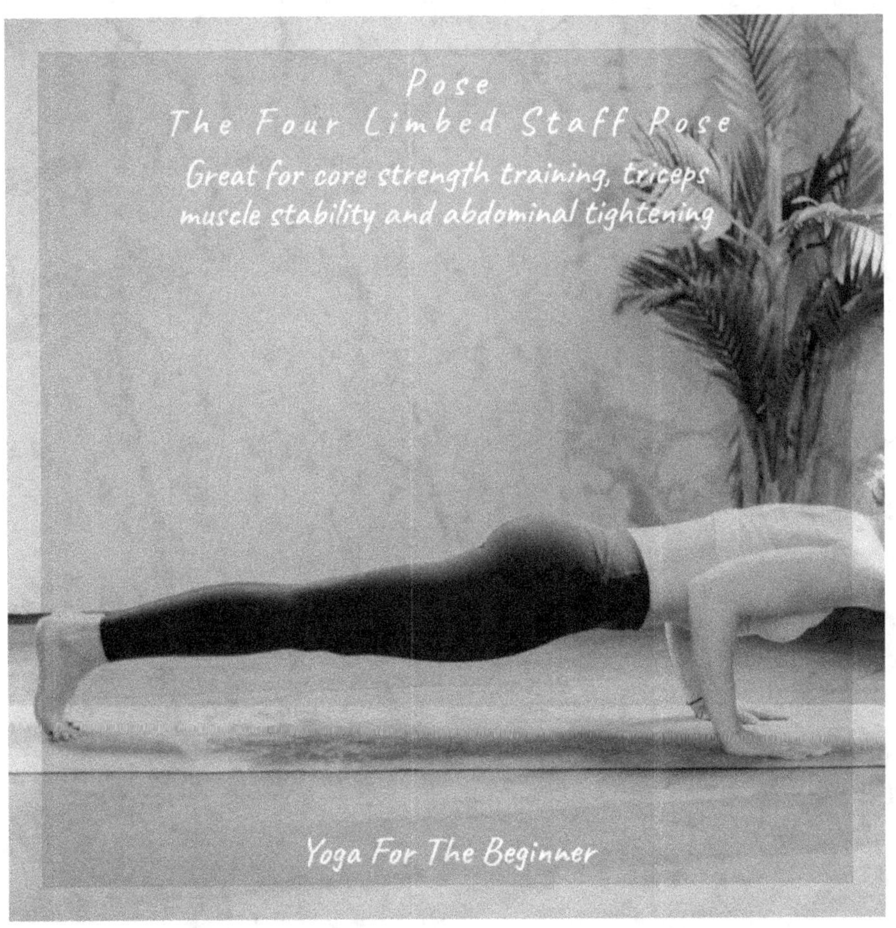

THE FOUR LIMBED STAFF POSE - (AKA) Chaturanga Dandasana

Number Six

THE SIDE PLANK POSE - (AKA) Vasisthasana

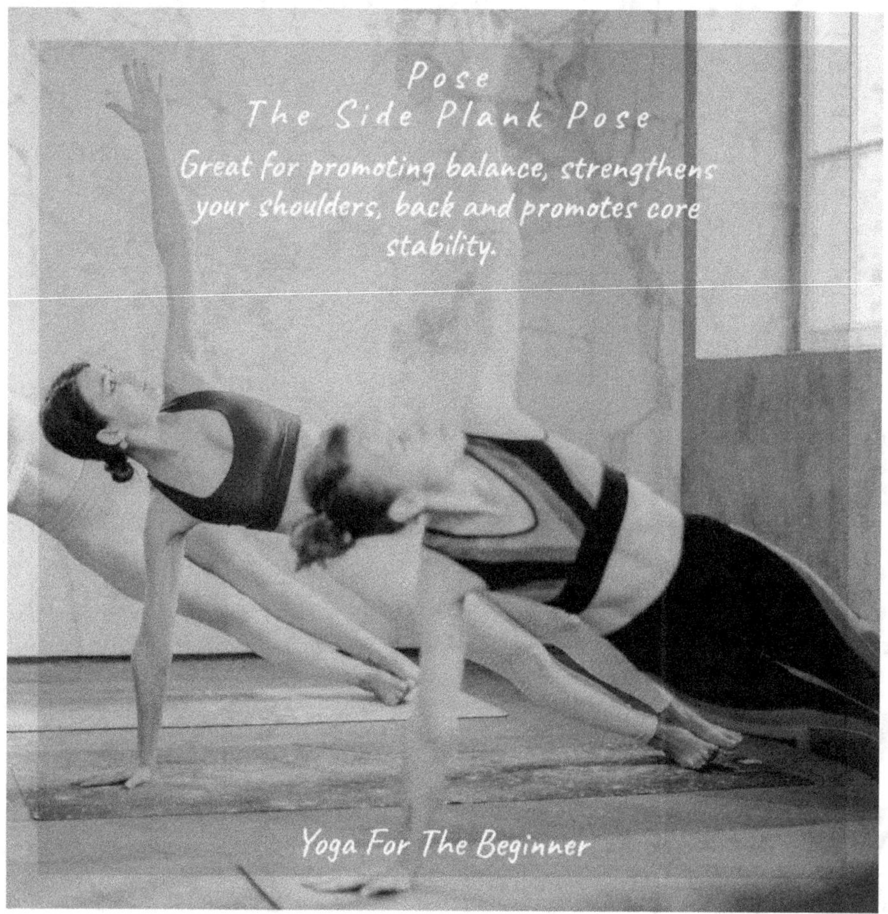

THE SIDE PLANK POSE - (AKA) Vasisthasana

Number Seven

THE EIGHT ANGLE POSE - (AKA) Astavakrasana

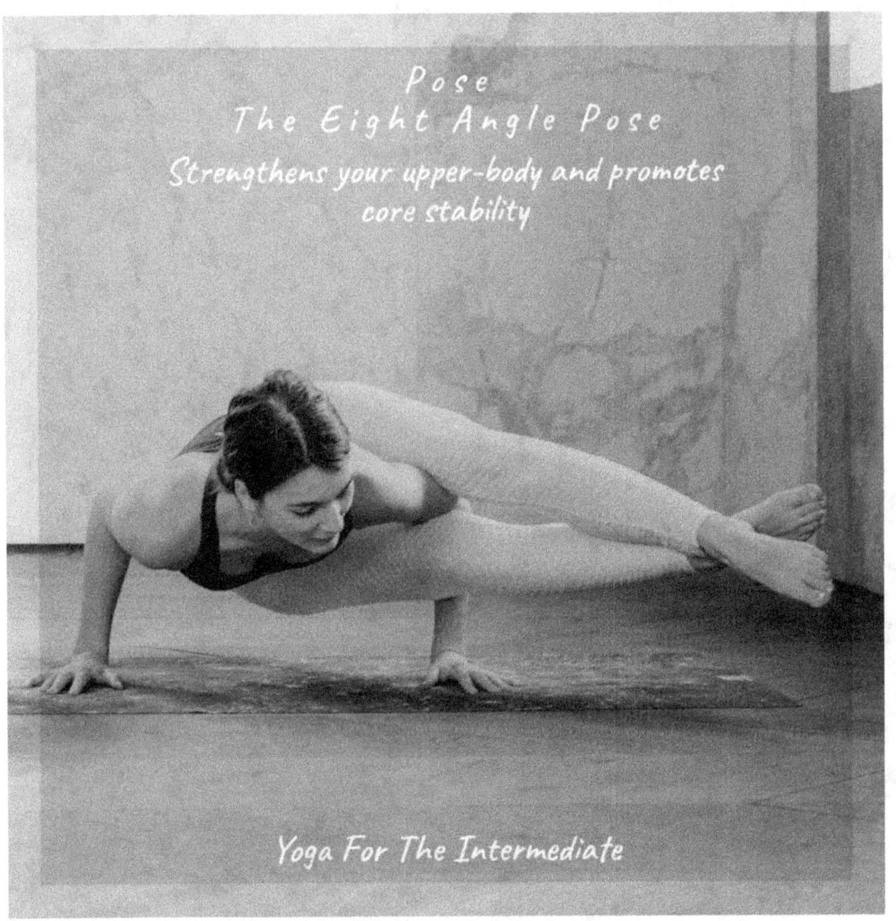

THE EIGHT ANGLE POSE - (AKA) Astavakrasana

Number Eight

THE WARRIOR I POSE - (AKA) Virabhadrasana I

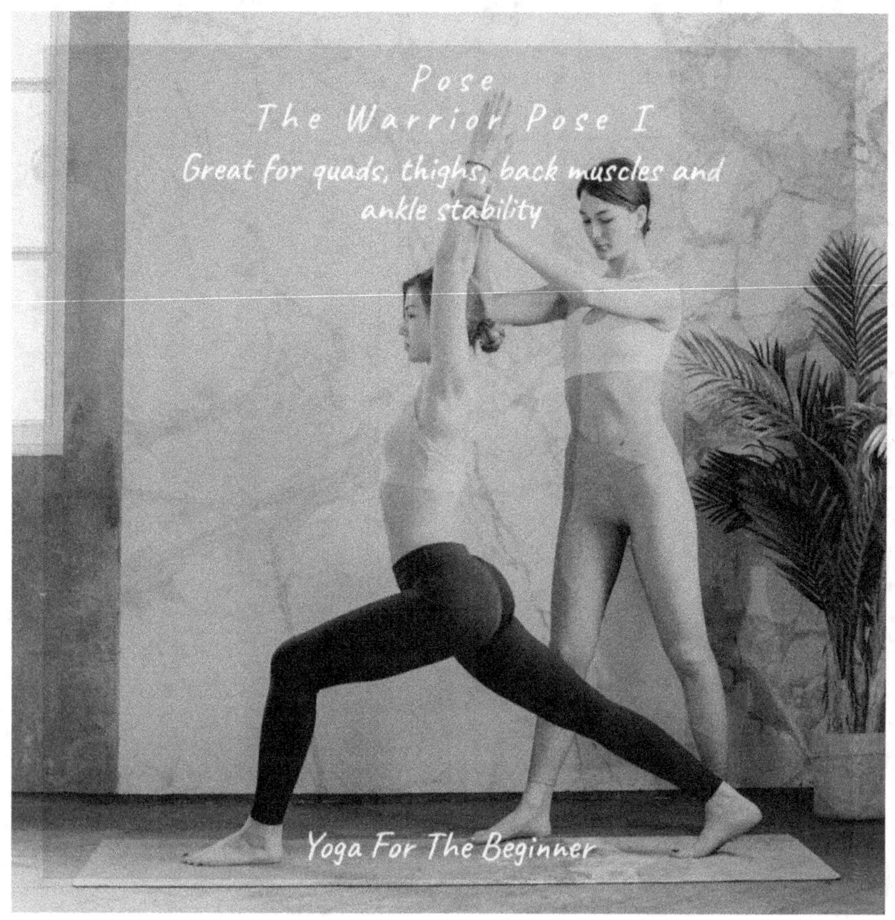

THE WARRIOR I POSE - (AKA) Virabhadrasana I

Number Nine

THE HANDSTAND POSE - (AKA) Adho Mukha Vrksasana

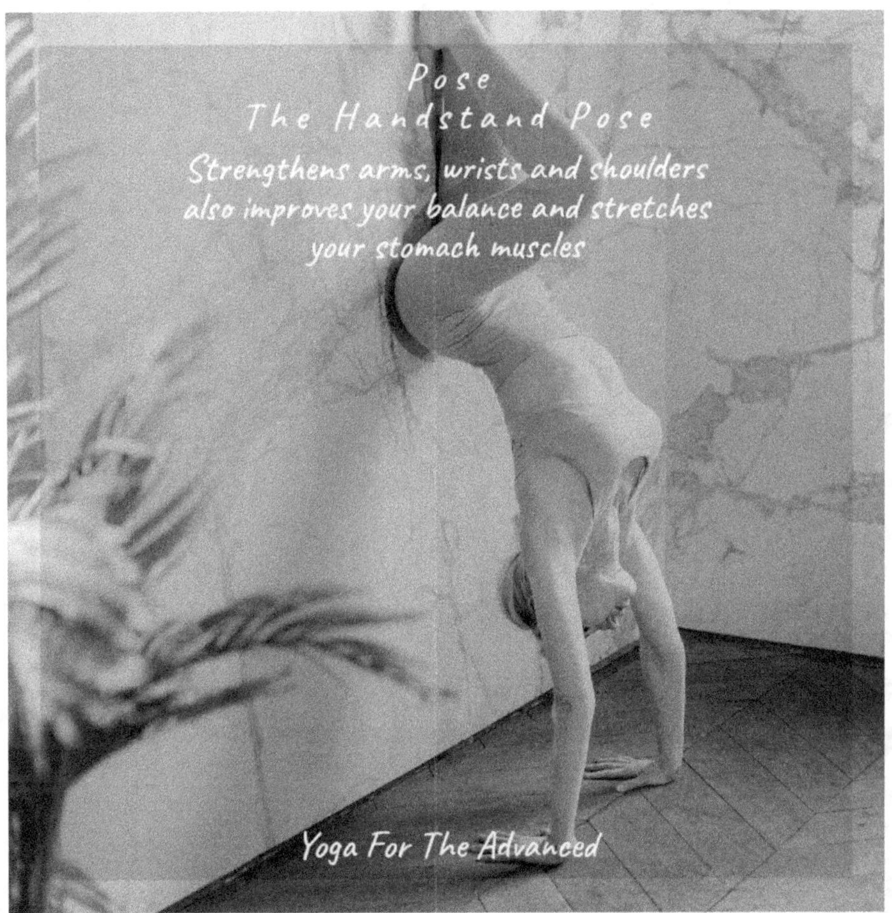

THE HANDSTAND POSE - (AKA) Adho Mukha Vrksasana

Number Ten

THE UPWARD FACING DOG POSE - (AKA)
Urdhva Mukha Svanasana

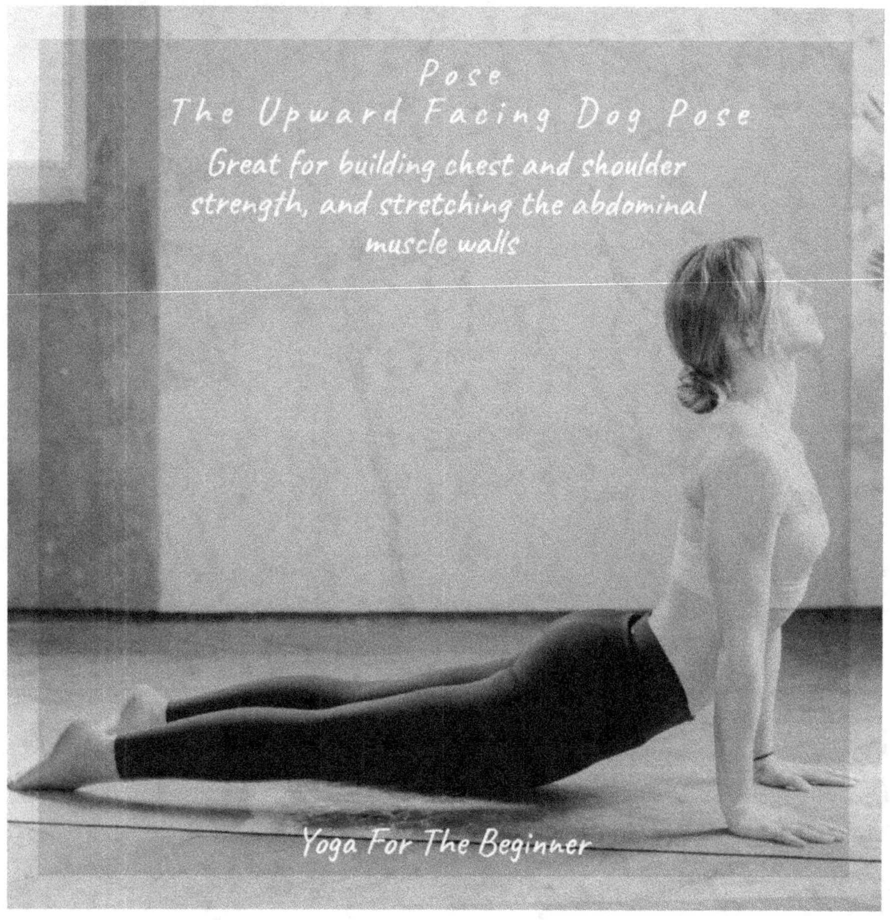

THE UPWARD FACING DOG POSE - (AKA) Urdhva Mukha Svanasana

In conclusion, one of the best things you can do for your mind, body, and spirit is to begin a yoga regime today.

Yoga as we have shown can be done anywhere, anytime on just about any flat stable surface, and with this knowledge now is the time for you to start developing your mind and body. I hope these pictures with included descriptions provide you with enough basic information to send you on your way to great health via yoga.

Remember yoga is not about attaining the perfect pose or posture, it's all about building confidence in your ability to perform the postures and poses safely and giving it your best shot, with the end result of you attaining the lasting mental, spiritual and physical health benefits of daily yoga exercise.

Namaste.

NAMASTE

Many people begin practicing yoga as a way to cope with feelings of anxiety, depression, pain or to lower their stress levels which are raised by everyday pressures. However, with this in mind, we can make good choices in what we choose to focus on within the practice of yoga. Yoga provides the bridge for clearing your mind, bringing you into a state of mindfulness, which in turn helps you deal with important life issues by way of focused breathing along with the learning of pose and posture control techniques designed to considerably lower your stress levels all without medication or other mood-enhancing supplements.

The benefits of yoga are not always visible right away. A person may see an improvement but the biggest impact is often in the long-term benefits of daily yoga practice. A decrease in feelings of anxiety is often the best benefit of the practice, and as we discussed there are certain types of poses that can increase the quality of life by lowering blood pressure and heart rate. However, there are many types of poses that can increase the quality of life by lowering anxiety.

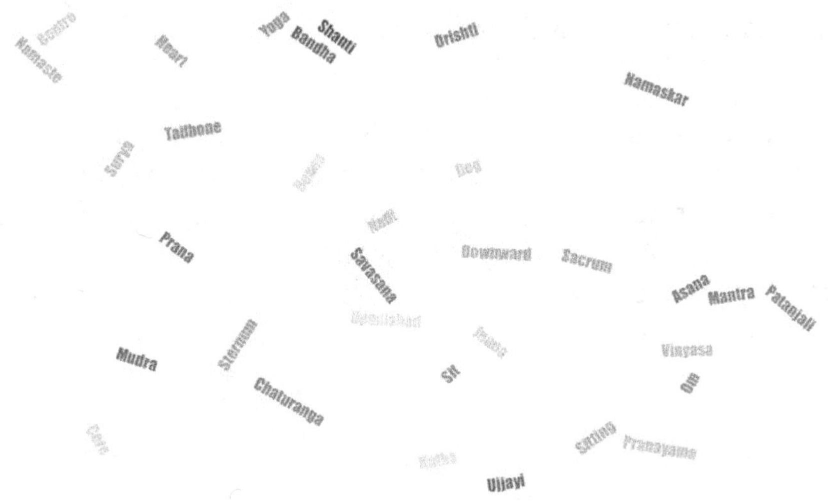

It is important to choose poses and instructions that will allow you to be fully aware of your breathing. With practice, we can learn to breathe slowly and fully. The benefits from each will increase together. This is a practice that can be practiced by anyone. It does not take an extraordinary amount of time but it takes a lot of practice to achieve results.

The type of pose is a very small factor. A person who practices is more likely to see long-term benefits than someone who does not. In the end, it all comes back to focusing on your breathing. If you take the time to focus on your breathing and relaxing your mind, the results will be seen more quickly. The long-term benefits which the practice of yoga delivers are immeasurable.

It is important to set aside time for daily practice. A person who does not take the time will miss out on the rewards. So if your life is crazy, hectic, stressful and out of control, then take the time, just a few minutes a day to do the yoga practice of your choosing and you will find the benefits of yoga will bring you directly into a calmer and more peaceful state of being.

I hope you practice and enjoy the extremely healthy benefits of yoga as I do, and whether your a novice, intermediate or advanced practitioner of Vinyasa, Hatha, Kundalini, Ashtanga, Bikram, Yin, Restorative, or Anusara yoga, I encourage you to continue the practice of yoga for the entirety of your life in order to improve the quality of your life each and every day.

Namaste.